Let's Look Together

An Interactive Picture Book
for People with Alzheimer's and
Other Forms of Memory Loss

by
Rae-Lynn Cebul Ziegler, OTR/L

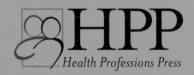

HPP
Health Professions Press

Baltimore • London • Sydney

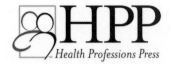

Health Professions Press, Inc.
Post Office Box 10624
Baltimore, Maryland 21285-0624
www.healthpropress.com

Interior and cover design by Joyce C. Weston Design.
Typeset by Joyce C. Weston.
Photography by Lynn Cañez, Third Floor Studios.
Manufactured in China by Jade Productions.

Library of Congress Cataloging-in-Publication Data

Ziegler, Rae-Lynn Cebul.
Let's look together : an interactive picture book for people
with Alzheimer's and other forms of memory loss / by
Rae-Lynn Cebul Ziegler.
  p. cm.
ISBN 978-1-932529-51-7 (pbk.)
1. Alzheimer's disease—Patients—Rehabilitation.
2. Memory disorders—Patients—Rehabilitation.
3. Picture books—Therapeutic use.
4. Occupational therapy. I. Title.
RC523.Z54 2009
616.8'3106—DC22

2009021878

British Library Cataloguing in Publication data are
available from the British Library.

"Sorrowful, yet always rejoicing"
(2 Corinthians 6:10)

To Mom, Alice C. Cebul, 1926–2005
In honor of her spirit of courage and grace,
and love of life and children.

To Dad, Raymond L. Cebul, 1924–2007
In honor of his love of his family and the
"spirit of the team."

To Barb Friedman, 1952–2004
In honor of sisterhood created, not born—a life
coach to me, a fellow OT, and the reason that
this book was nurtured to publication.

Contents

Introduction

This book has a very basic purpose. It is intended to be used as an activity that encourages meaningful interaction between a person living with a cognitive disability and a caregiver, family member, or other individual who wishes to make an emotional or cognitive connection with that person. Hopefully the pleasant mood of the time spent together over this book will stay with the person even if he or she cannot remember what you did together.

One of the beauties of this book is that it presents a *failure-free* activity that can be individualized in unlimited and creative ways that succeed in the moment and honor the integrity of the connection. At its best, this book is a tool to help connect with the person with mental (cognitive) impairment wherever he or she is at any given moment, and in so doing it becomes a bridge to the abilities that remain and are not lost.

The book can be used with anyone, regardless of gender, ethnic background, age, or stage of physical or emotional ability.

Background

This book has evolved from a personal to a professional tool. It started as a way to connect with my own mother, who was diagnosed with Alzheimer's disease. At the point when Mom had lost most of her ability to talk coherently and to express what she might be thinking, it seemed that she still generally understood what I was saying but was unable to speak back to me. Communication abilities can break down on both incoming (*receptive aphasia*) and outgoing (*expressive aphasia*) levels. My mother, who had always been very articulate, appeared to have developed expressive aphasia, which prevented her from making her thoughts known.

As an occupational therapist, I was better equipped than most people to think of things to do with Mom and to be therapeutically creative with her, but even I began to struggle with the limitations of our interactions. I desperately wanted to preserve our deep connections as mother and daughter. I conceived of a book that we could share together. I liked the idea that we could sit side by side and feel each other's presence.

The Theory

Putting my occupational training to work, I turned to the theories of A. Jean Ayres, an occupational therapist with advanced training in the neurosciences, normal child development, and adaptive behavior, who developed the theory of sensory integration in the early 1960s. She used the theory with children who were experiencing learning deficits. I use it in this book.

Dr. Ayres looked at how people use all the information collected through the five senses: taste/**gustatory**, hearing/**auditory**, smell/**olfactory**, touch/**tactile**, sight/**visual**; the perception of body parts and movements through muscles, joints, and tendons/**proprioception**; and the perception of gravity and movement through space/**vestibular**. Her concept of sensory integration describes the process by which the body's central nervous system (the brain and spinal cord) *takes in* information from the environment and then *organizes and processes* the sensations for meaningful use in our daily occupation, whether we are at play or learning or fulfilling roles, such as mother or doctor. Virtually everything we do and every skill we use is the product of sensory integration, which is a theory of brain–behavior relationships (Bundy, Lane & Murray, 2002).

When the nervous system perceives sensory information, a very complex, synchronized, logical, and sequential process must occur before we can react to the sensation and respond meaningfully and appropriately, whether it is smiling at a friendly greeting or snatching our hand away from a hot surface. This process is analogous to getting an e-mail:

1. *You've got mail.* Your body perceives an incoming message (sensory registration).

2. *Who is it from?* Your body decides whether the information is useful and what priority to assign to it (sensory engagement and regulation).

3. *What do I do with this information?* Your body decides if it wants to read or file the information (memory capacity).

4. *Reply.* You decide to respond to the information in a way that is meaningful to you (behavioral response [e.g., an action such as speaking, pointing, smiling, frowning, turning away from the stimulus]).

Through a multitude of neuronal connections, the brain sorts the sensory experience and determines whether to discard it, use it immediately, file it for later use as a long-term memory (e-mail files), or place it in a short-term memory file for new learning to take place.

Ayres' theory contends that "learning is dependent on the ability to take in and process sensation from movement and the environment and use it to plan and organize behavior" (Bundy, Lane & Murray, 2002). Each individual responds to information based on his or her own unique experiences and emotions, individual interests, and need for the information. Additionally, abilities such as concentration, attention span, emotional responsiveness, coordination of body movements, and language or speech also influence a person's response. Diseases such as Alzheimer's or genetic conditions that affect cognitive abilities, such as Down syndrome or autism, interfere with these abilities and, thus, with the behavioral response to stimuli. The result is sensory integration dysfunction. Clinicians educated in sensory integration theory argue that enhancing the sensory environment of individuals who have processing challenges will help them achieve a more organized behavioral response and improve their sensory integration capability (Bundy, Lane & Murray, 2002).

According to learning theories, four key factors impact human learning retention:

- *Repetition.* Repeated actions can be thought of as "practice opportunities."

- *Multisensory information.* Experiencing multiple body sensations (e.g., sight, sound, movement, touch) stimulates brain activity and increases a person's ability to learn and retain information (e.g., learning the alphabet through a song). Note that each person has a preferred sensory system for learning, but if one sensory system fails to work efficiently, another one attempts to compensate.

- *Intensity.* The strength or intensity of a sensory experience has been found to increase the brain's ability to learn, retain, and respond (e.g., an exaggerated facial expression, a loud or whispered voice, a comment accompanied by a physical touch on the hand).

- *Frequency.* How frequently a person experiences a sensation impacts individual learning ability.

All four of these factors are seen to one degree or another throughout this book and can be used while interacting with the person with cognitive impairment to enhance the sensory integration and sensory engagement process.

How This Book Benefits Those with Cognitive Impairments

By design, the photographs in this book are not accompanied by words that dictate how to use or interpret them. The shared activity of looking through the pages of the book carries no sense of right or wrong, which encourages the person with a cognitive deficit to freely share his or her responses to the photographs. Being encouraged to respond to the photographs in any way that naturally arises produces a sense of mastery and positive feelings that are too often eroded through the course of Alzheimer's disease.

The concept of this book worked very effectively with my mother, but I also wanted to see if the collection of photographs I had chosen, sequenced, and strategically placed on each page were equally effective with others at various stages of dementia. I conducted a research study with residents of an assisted living facility in Wake Forest, North Carolina. The results of this study appear on pages 55–57.

Each person in the study, regardless of the varied backgrounds, was willing to become engaged in a meaningful way with the person who offered them the book as an activity, albeit for different individual periods of time (on average, for approximately 15 minutes). Each person made good eye contact with the photos in the book. The majority of participants were assessed as having had a positive experience, responding in a recognizable physical or verbal way through gestures, such as smiling or laughing, or through the use of words (e.g., "look"), phrases (e.g., "well, there you are!"), or expressions (e.g., "how cute").

Some of the important features I built into the book include the following:

Subject

- People respond to the human face and to the facial configuration of the eyes, nose, and mouth—an innate response that's observable from infancy onward.

- Pictures of children are featured in the book because infants and children seem to provoke an almost universal response, whether or not a person has a child, is young or old, or male or female, and regardless of socio-economic or racial background.

Format

- Photographs, as opposed to drawings, evoke a stronger emotional relationship and interaction because they are based in reality.

- The photographs show children who the person is not expected to know, removing any strain associated with identifying them, thereby creating an emotional distance that is therapeutically beneficial.

Visibility

- Images on each page are simple and clear with high contrast for easy processing.

- Primary colors provide strong visual stimulation.

Interest

- The photos are strategically placed on each page to create unexpected variety and visual interest.

- Variety is also created with children of differing ages and who are performing different activities.

Engagement

- Photos produce direct eye contact with the viewer.
- Basic human emotions are portrayed—happiness, sadness, anger, surprise, fear, disgust—and can lead to cognitive and physical responses, including mimicking an expression or producing a vocal or verbal reaction.
- Activities are portrayed that stimulate sensory memory (hearing, taste, smell) and activate the pleasures and sensations experienced from them.
- Children are inherently spontaneous and playful, which draws the viewer into the photo.

The goal of each turn of the page is to "wake up" the brain and get it interacting and responding to the photograph in a way that can lead to an interactive relationship with the caregiver.

Of course, everyone has good days and bad days. There may be days—or even moments or times of the day—when the person with cognitive disability cannot pay attention and respond well to the photos in this book. There may be days when this same person experiences no feelings and offers no responses to the photos at all. For me, growing to accept each day for what it was for my mother, with grace, became a healing process for both me and, I believe, for her. My hope is the same for you as it was for me and my mother: that you can use this book to become emotionally present to the best of your ability for someone with cognitive disability, so that both of you can feel connected and bonded in that moment.

At times, your partner will look at only some of the photos, but at other times may look at them all. Sometimes with my mother, I would immediately start the book over again, and it would seem that her brain had warmed up and she could pay attention much better! You may share the book just one time or several times in a day. Each time is likely to be a fresh, new experience, especially when the focus of using the book is on being together and using the relationship to stimulate the brain.

In the following section, you will find a collection of tips for constructively using the book and communicating with a person with cognitive disability. The most important advice of all, however, is never to allow the person who is viewing the book to feel that the activity is childish. At all times, honor the life experience and the integrity of the person with whom you are experiencing the book.

In the end, let your imagination be your guide with this book. It is meant to be a pleasurable and open-ended adventure!

User's Guide

Use the following tips to increase your success when sharing this book with someone with cognitive disability.

Tip 1: The one-on-one, side-by-side nature of this activity should help to increase the person's capacity to focus during the activity.

Tip 2: Be aware of what is going on in the environment around you. Don't overload a person's nervous system with external sensory information when he or she isn't able to regulate or process the stimuli effectively. (Consider how your body feels when you are tired at the end of a long day, and how hard it can be to tolerate too much noise or activity.) Use common sense in selecting where to look at the book and choose a location without excessive noise (e.g., people talking in the immediate area) and without people or activity that might be visually distracting.

Tip 3: In general, ask open-ended questions (e.g., "What kind of pies do you like?" as opposed to "Is she eating a cherry or apple pie?"). The goal is to ask questions that have no right or wrong answers. Use the photos to prompt conversation or to trigger a memory that facilitates talking.

Tip 4: If the person is not able to remain relatively calm and focused, you can try to work your way gently and slowly to an appropriate conversation. Everyone has emotional defenses that they use to protect themselves when feeling vulnerable. If the caregiver attempts to go outside of the person's defense mechanisms—too much, too fast—it is natural for that person to shut down, close up, or otherwise retreat in some way to regain a sense of internal balance. Recognize and acknowledge that the person might be feeling overwhelmed.

Tip 5: Encourage taking a break from looking at the photographs. Stretch or have both of you move and gently shake your arms to wake up your bodies. This break is another source of sensory input that can be reorganizing—much like when you are tired from reading or sitting and watching television and you get up to eat something, get a cold drink, or chew a piece of flavorful gum.

Secrets for Successful Communication

When you sit down to look at this book with a person with cognitive disability, try to follow these communication guidelines. Some may be intuitive and natural for you, while others may require thought, patience, and loving discipline.

- At all times preserve the dignity of the person with whom you are using the book. Extend compassion and acceptance to the person, who might be feeling alone, confused, fearful, and frustrated.

- Treat the person with integrity. Recognize that the person is an adult who has fulfilled a meaningful role in this world (e.g., mother, brother, teacher). Don't treat an adult with a cognitive impairment like a child!

- Place yourself close enough to the person so that he or she cannot only hear you, but also intimately sense your presence.

- Speak slowly, clearly, and calmly to assist with the processing of the information you are providing to the person (this does not mean you need to speak loudly).

- Be aware of what your body is saying about your true intentions. Consciously use eye contact, body language, the tone and inflection of your voice, and physical proximity to communicate positive regard for the person.

- Deliver simple messages, one at a time. Short, concrete comments or questions are easiest to process (e.g., "Smell that rose!" "Yum, ice cream!" "Is he happy?").

- Use a multisensory approach:
  - Show the picture (visual cue).
  - Say something to elicit a verbal reply (auditory cue).
  - Touch the person's hand or arm, or lead his or her hand to the page (tactile cue).
  - Wait for a response (registration/processing/response time).
  - Repeat the sensory sequence if you get no response.
  - Once the person seems to have lost interest in a photo after multiple cues, turn the page and try a fresh image and topic.

- Do not race through the book. Go slowly and take your lead from the person with cognitive disability. Allow time for the person to respond to what he or she has seen, heard, or felt. The person's processing time may be slower than you anticipate it to be.

- Recognize that behavior can change over the course of the disease.

- Learn what you can about the individual's abilities. Try to lovingly and realistically match your communication and responses to these abilities. In particular, awareness of time and abstract ideas will be affected and impaired.

- Be prepared for different responses from day to day. Every day is a different day, and each time of the day may be different from the hour before it!

- Verbalize emotions and sensations that the person may experience from a photo. You can comment, "You seem like you might be feeling sad when you look at the baby in this picture" or "Look how soft the baby's skin seems!" or "Wow, that person's hair is curly!" Create opportunities to discuss emotions and sensations that might be felt.

- Be positive and supportive of any comment the person makes. For example, say "Tell me about that" or simply "Tell me more." If the photo stimulates a memory for the person, that's wonderful. If it does not, let the person talk about whatever topic or reaction arises in the moment.

- Repeat some of the person's own words, adding emphasis, an exclamation, or turning the comment into a question directed back to the person. For example, if the person says, "That boy looks happy," you could ask, "Do you think that boy looks really happy?"

- If you don't get a response to a prompt, try rephrasing or restating what you have said. For example, "What's he eating?" "Is he eating something?" "What do you think he's doing?"

- If the person is agitated or distressed, try to identify what factors might be causing the distress and deal with them (e.g., is the person hungry, constipated, fearful, hallucinating, or overstimulated?). Once the person's distress is addressed, try to work the conversation to a more positive place. If the person does not become engaged or continues to be agitated, do not force him or her to participate!

- Avoid whispering or talking about the person in front of him or her. Don't assume the person has a hearing or comprehension problem.

- Have and use a sense of humor. It can have wonderful therapeutic advantages!

- Be open to whatever the person tells you he or she sees in the picture. Encourage an attitude of curiosity. Unexpected feelings and conversations can emerge and produce a wonderful sense of having shared a bit of meaningful time and relationship together.

Use the following questions as a guide for ways to engage the person in an exchange about the photographs.

What is the child doing?

What do you see?

Tell me about this picture.

That little girl/boy sure is having fun!

Are there colors that you like in this picture?

What is the child eating? It looks like it might be cold/hot/sticky.

What do you like to eat?

How is this child feeling?

How are you feeling today?

How does the picture of this child make you feel?

Did your own son/daughter ever do this? [If you know that the person had children.]

That mother looks like she loves her child—what do you think?

Can you make a happy face like this child?

Can you make your arms look like his or hers?

How do you look when you are angry?

Let's make up a story about what is happening in this photo!

Tell me about this picture. Can you tell me more?

That girl looks really surprised! Does she look surprised to you?

Let's smell that rose! Does it remind you of your garden?

Hello? Who's on the phone? [Mimic behavior.]

Uh-oh! or Oh, no!

Here's what I like—look at the soft hair on that child! [Point to something that you like in the picture.]

Another approach to looking at the pictures is to incorporate cognitive concepts, such as the following:

What colors do you see?

How many fingers do you count?

Is the picture large or small?

Do you think this child is a boy or girl?

How old do you think the person in this photograph is?

Do you think that the baby is soft or rough?

Is the ice cream cold or hot?

Finally, you can make your own statements or observations about a photo. For example, you might state what you see in the photo or how it makes you feel ("I loved ice cream when I was a child!"). You can also simply say, "Hmmm" or "Oh, look!" or "How silly that child is being." Your comments will model for the person ways to respond or will validate what the person might be sensing but can't express in his or her own words.

Using the Book with Groups

The original intent and design of *Let's Look Together* was for one-on-one, side-by-side interaction, but it can also be used with groups. When working with a small group, you must take into account the following activity components:

Environment. Before starting, consider the whole environment. Is the lighting too light or dark? Is surrounding noise quiet or distracting? Is there too much visual stimulation (lots of posters, hanging objects, filled tables)? Are there distracting fragrances or odors from a nearby source? Look at the positioning of everyone in the group: Are people in their chairs upright and secure, with feet supported? Can they see you from where they are? Are they next to someone with whom they are compatible?

Group size. Don't try to use the book with too large a group. Test it with a small number of people and find the group size that works best and that you are comfortable with.

Group composition and dynamics. Depending on the nature of the activity, decide who the individual participants will be. You may need to make adjustments for their personal qualities and characteristics, such as temperaments and compatibility, level of cognitive ability, language skills, mobility or physical limitations, and visual or hearing impairments.

Task analysis. This is the process of breaking down an activity into single "units" of activity to determine how to successfully achieve each "unit." For example, can the group or person concentrate for 2 minutes to take a turn in a game? Can the person pick up dice and toss them? Can the person look at you and then at the page to answer a question in some way?

Activity selection. The choice and success of an activity will depend heavily on the task-analysis process.

Use the suggestions that follow as a springboard for thinking of your own imaginative ideas for using this book as an activity.

10

Just add music. Select one or more of the photographs and match some music to them. Adding music may encourage individuals in the group to express their reactions to the photos through body movement, singing or humming, laughing, or mimicking a facial expression. You could even use musical and rhythmic instruments and let participants create their own musical interpretation (beware of using too many instruments and becoming too loud and confusing).

Showing a photo along with accompanying music can encourage people to talk. Music taps into many areas of the brain, including the language centers. Not only language, but also memory, emotion, and movement can be stimulated by music because of how music integrates the nervous system by using many different parts of the brain.

Get dramatic. Let the photos serve as inspiration for a short improvisational skit. Have staff perform while explaining—in a simple, direct way—what they are creating, or have them use only actions and no words (pantomime). For some groups, the actions alone may be the "just right" experience, because too many stimuli—words, actions, colors, group dynamics—may be overwhelming for those who have lower cognitive abilities.

Create a story. If you have a group whose language skills are relatively intact, try placing three of the photos side by side and asking everyone to make up a story about them. The story may not end up making a lot of sense, but social, language, and cognitive skills will be used in the process. The focus should be on having fun together!

Play a game. Have the group decide who is the oldest and who is the youngest in pictures that you select from the book. Choose two, three, or possibly up to five photos, depending on the participants' cognitive abilities. Maybe the group can put all the people from the book in some kind of order relative to their ages.

Play a matching game based on emotions or activities. Using images from other sources, find pictures that show various emotions or activities. Give Bingo chips to participants and ask them to place a chip on the face of the child in the book who is sad, for example, or who is eating.

Have participants bring in family photographs of children (grandchildren, their own children as youngsters, or even themselves as youngsters); then try to match their own photos to pictures in the book (e.g., by age, by activity, by gender, by expression).

Reference

Bundy, Lane & Murray (2002). *Sensory integration theory and practice, second edition*. Philadelphia: F. A. Davis Company.

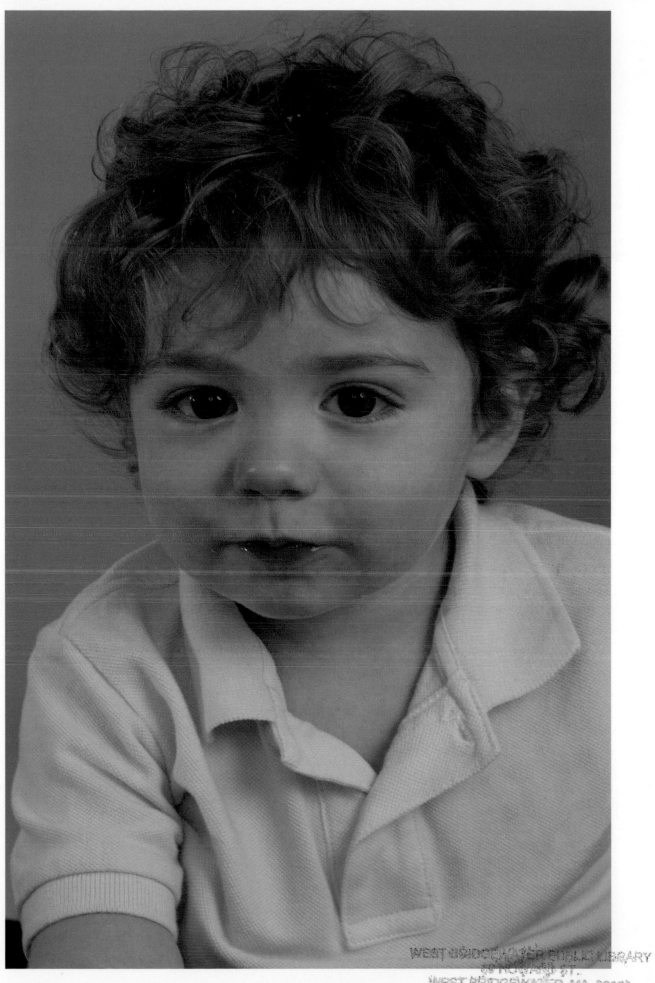

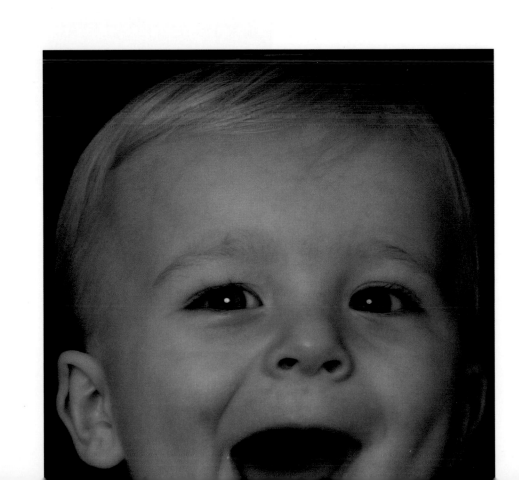

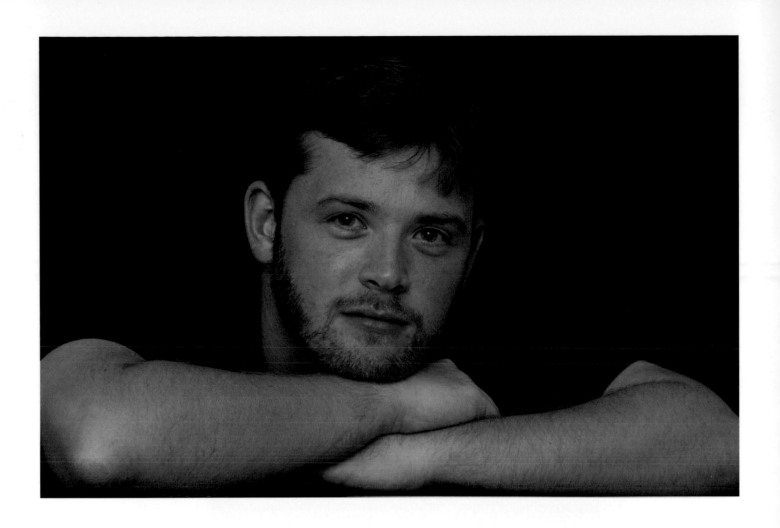

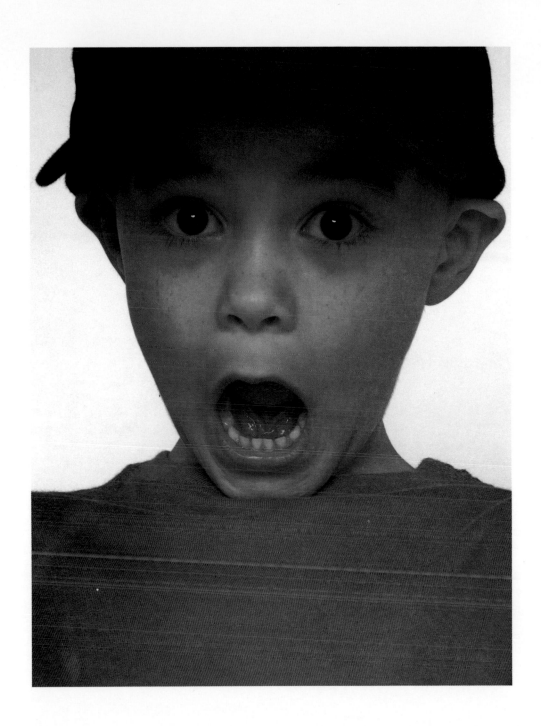

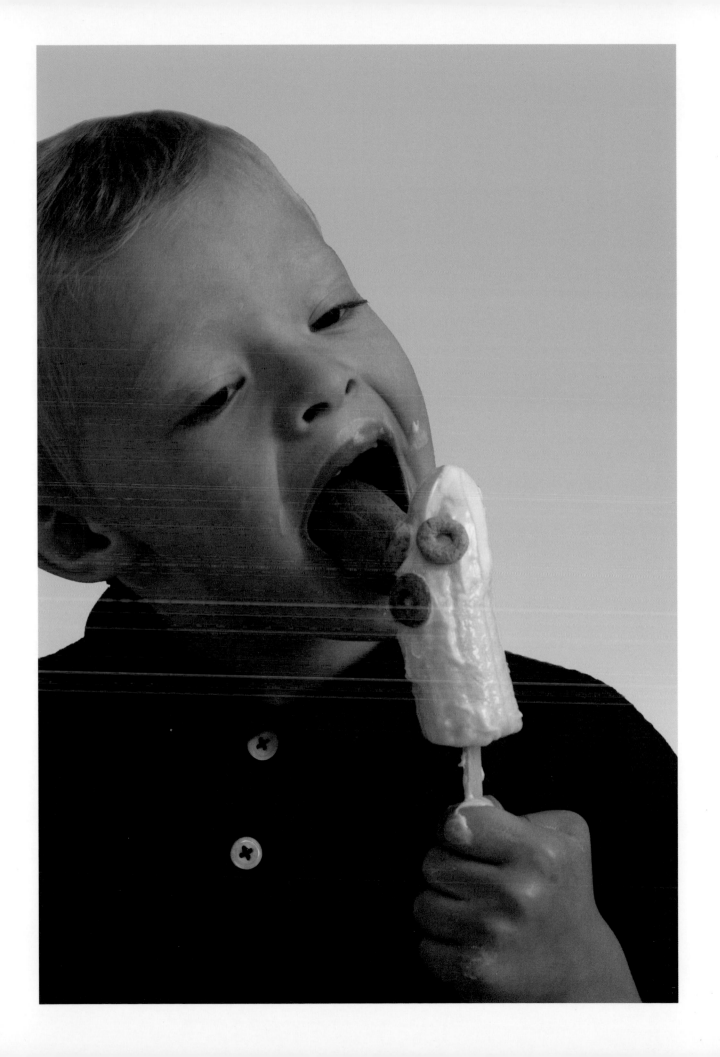

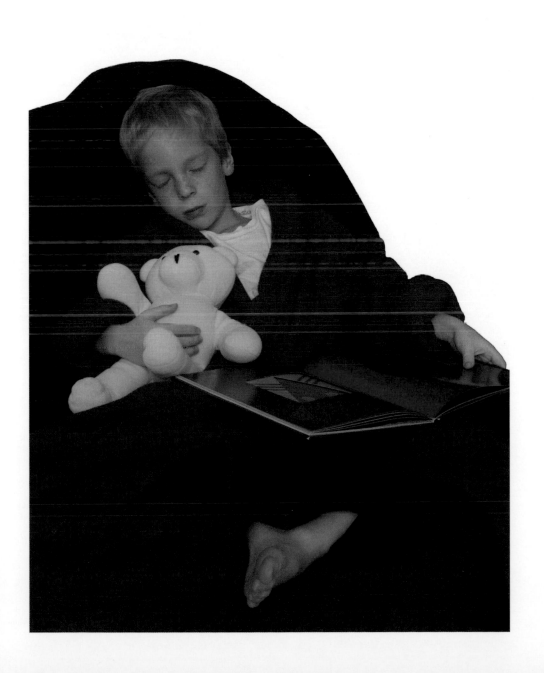

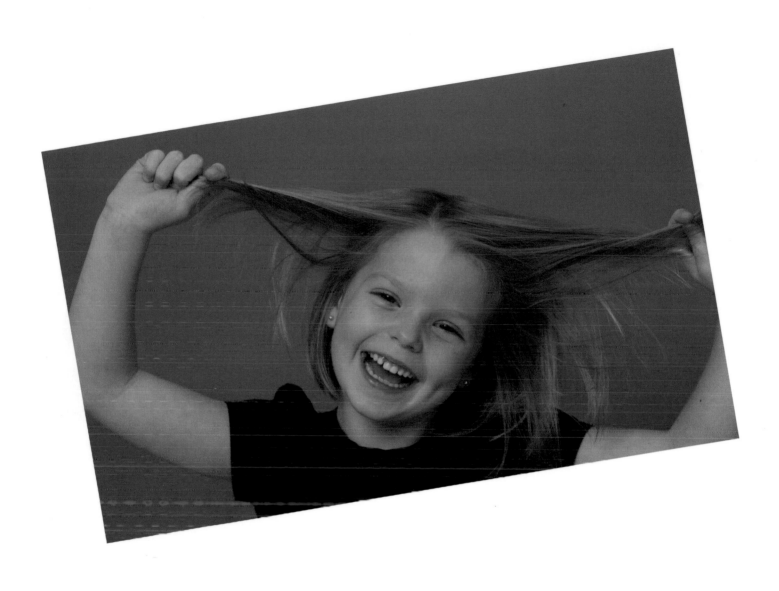

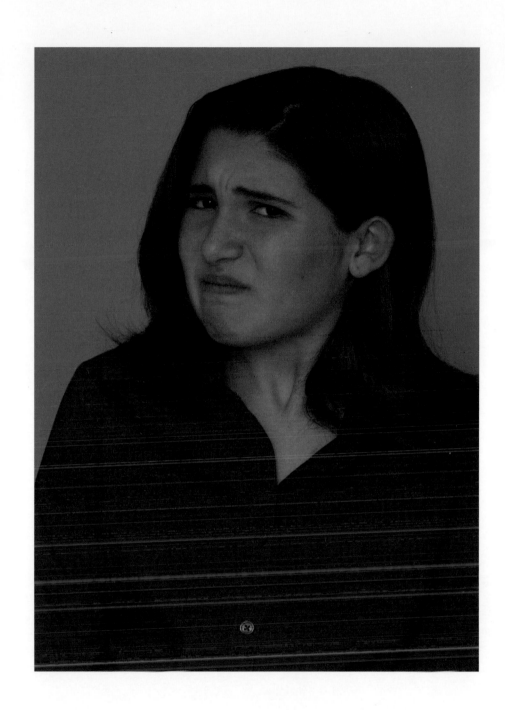

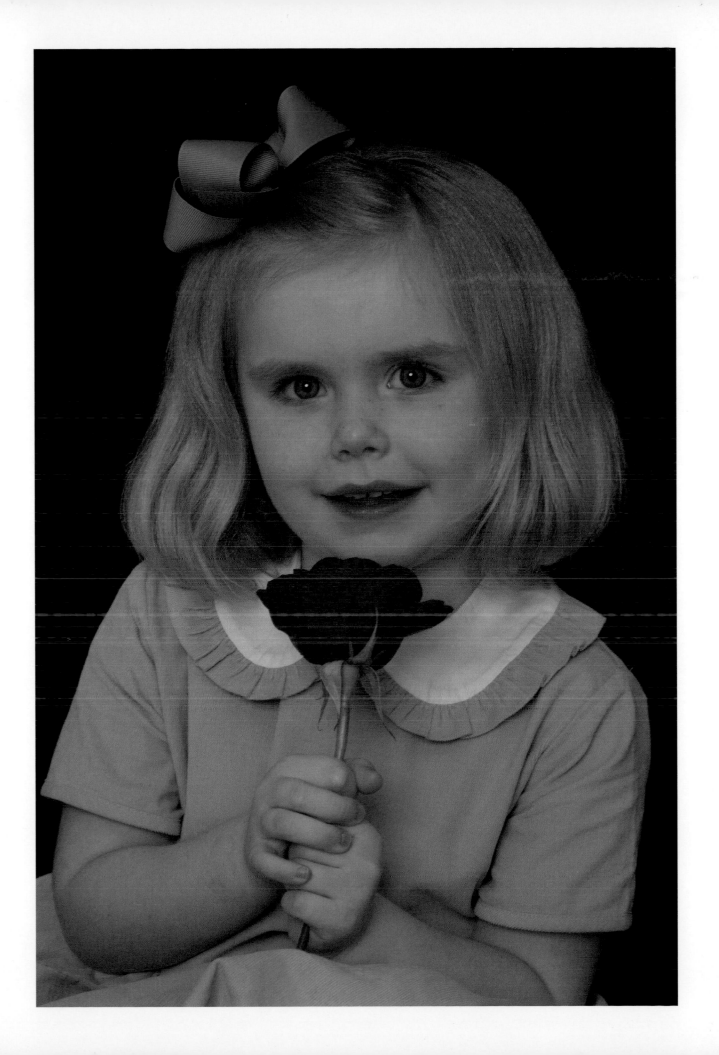

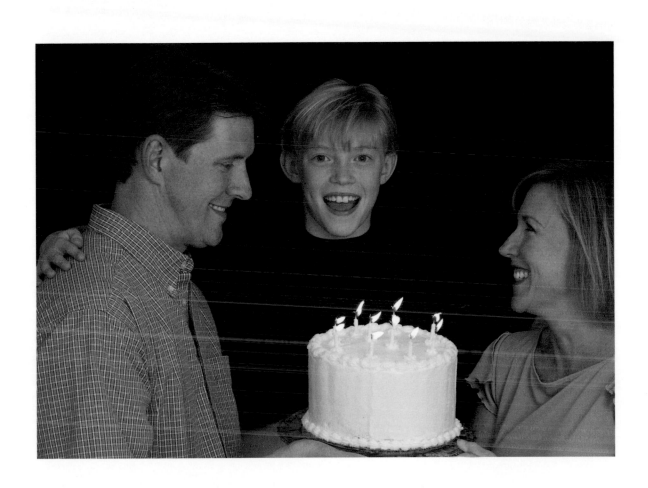

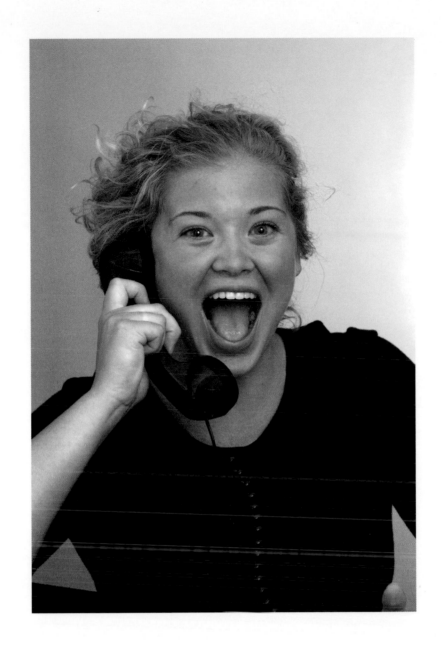

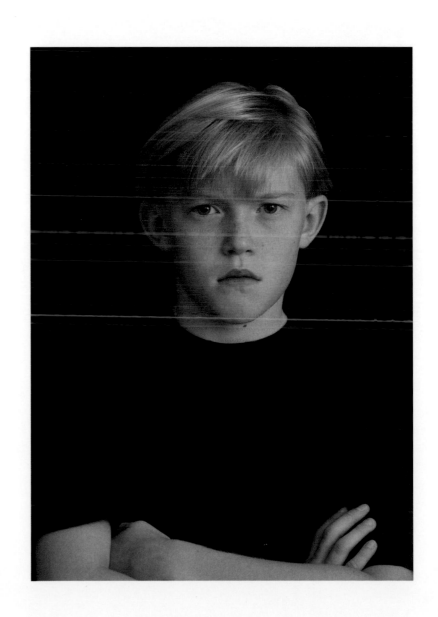

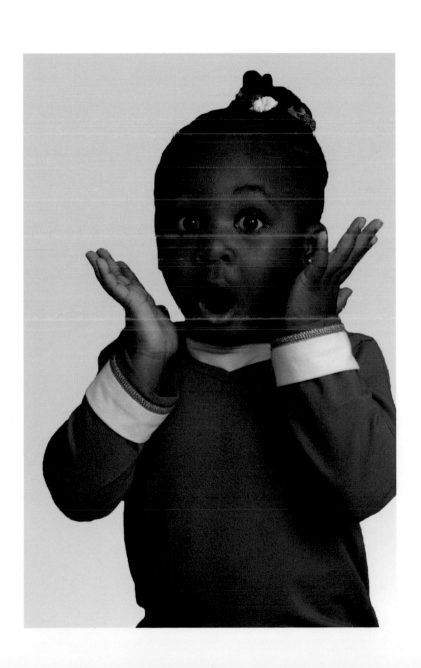

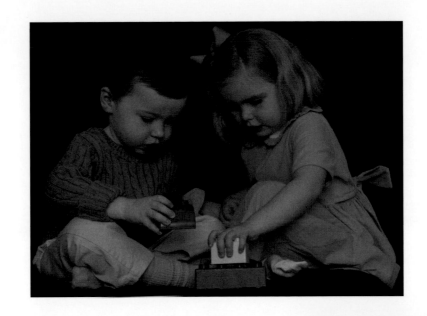

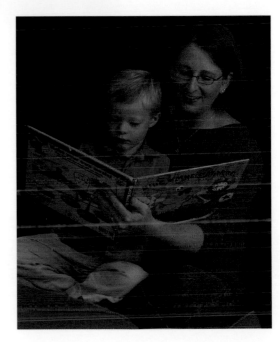

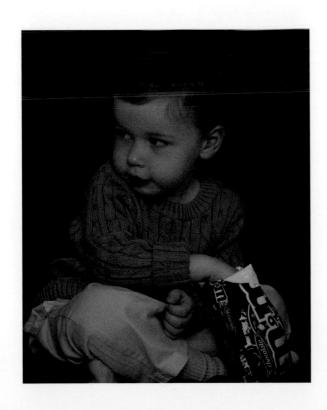

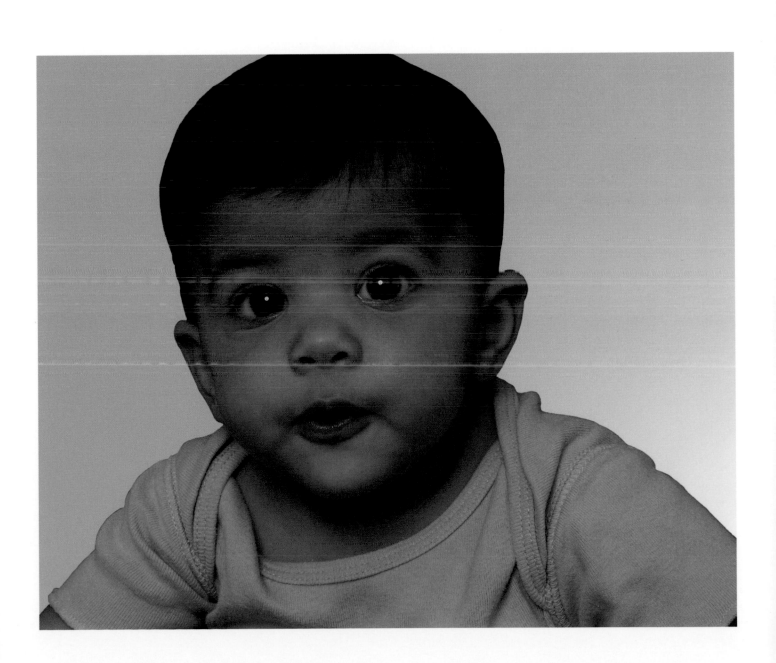

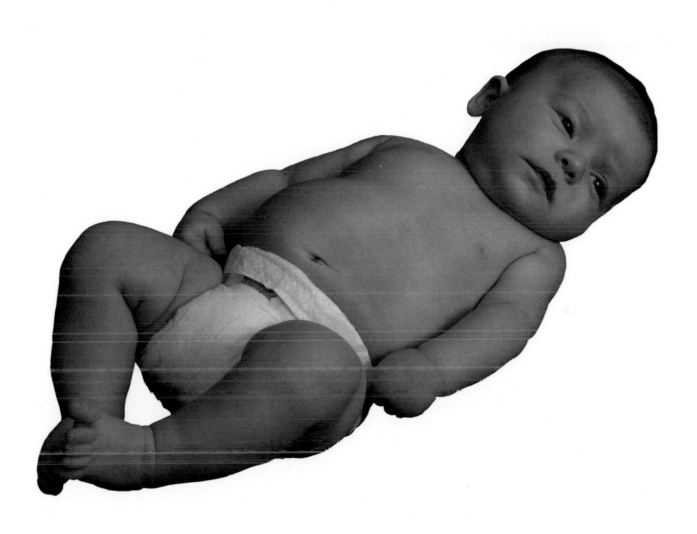

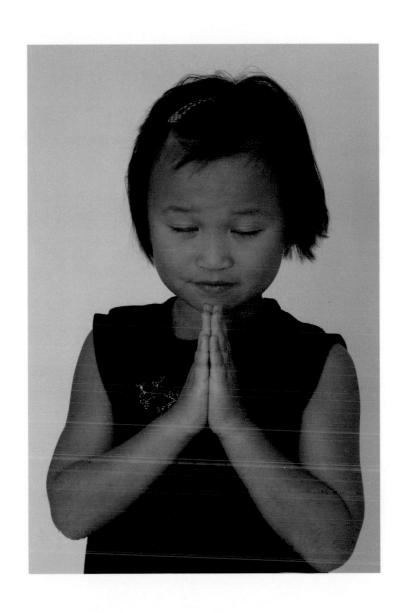

Appendix

I first developed this book concept for use with my mother, but then I wanted to see if it was equally effective with others who have dementia. So I conducted a research study using a 25-photo prototype book with residents at an assisted living facility in Wake Forest, North Carolina.

A group of 13 older adults was selected by the Divisional Memory Care Specialist from the facility's dementia unit. Participants were chosen for variety in gender, age, level of dementia, and socio-economic, racial, and ethnic background. The book was presented to each participant in the same place (a room relatively free of noise and traffic) and in the same manner (residents were seated immediately next to the researcher, who held the book within their view). A second researcher recorded behavioral responses, noting any physical or verbal expressions prompted by each photo.

Recorded facial expressions or general responses. These included frowning, sad expression, look of amazement, broad smile, lit-up face, flat affect, pensive and studied gaze, general lack of interest, no engagement with the photograph at all, simple visual exploration of the page, mimicry of the photograph, or response only to a verbal prompt.

Use of hands. In general, participants did not initiate turning the pages of the book. One participant took the book from the facilitator, a few touched the pages as if to study the photo, some did not use their hands at all the entire time, a nominal few pointed at features in the pictures, and very few responded to hand-over-hand guidance or a verbal prompt to initiate and follow through with page turning. One person, when left alone, turned the pages independently, but otherwise it appeared that the ability to initiate page turning was difficult.

Body language. The majority of participants were calm, still, docile, content, and engaged; some were animated, while others demonstrated a flat affect and lack of engagement through their body language. One participant was agitated prior to sitting down to look at the book and was challenging to get engaged by the facilitator or to get focused on the photos. This participant's body language could be described as "not calm" and tending to move "away from" the activity.

Recorded vocal sounds. These included giggling, laughing, making "raspberries," exclaiming "oh" (frequent), and attempting to mimic a sound suggested by the photograph. Vocal sounds were defined as anything that was not an articulated word.

Recorded words. The level of cognitive disability was reflected in the fullness (or lack thereof) of what was literally spoken. The range of words or comments included: "Eating it and loving it!"; "I hope nobody bothers me"; "I feel sad too"; "He's mad as can be!"; "In his teens—smil'in"; "A lot of fingers there"; "Don't care about it—take it"; "Oh, look at her"; "What is that here?"; "Happy child"; "Memories"; "Oh, darl'in"; "I love you." At times the words did not relate to the photograph.

As noted in the introduction (p. 4), each person in the study became engaged in a meaningful way with the book as an activity. Individual durations of engagement are noted in the chart on page 56, along with specific behavioral responses. The average time spent engaged with the book was approximately 15 minutes. Each person made good eye contact with the photos in the book, and nearly everyone (12/13 persons) was viewed as having had a positive experience by virtue of responding in recognizable physical or verbal ways, such as smiling, laughing, or uttering a word (e.g., "look"), phrase (e.g., "well, there you are!"), or expression (e.g., "how cute"). The importance of taking time to initiate trust and develop some relationship with the participant was seen as imperative for the success and quality of the book-viewing experience.

Research Data: Reactions to Photography Book Prototype

Participant	# of pictures that elicited a positive response	# of pictures that elicited a negative response	# of pictures that elicited a neutral response	# of pictures that elicited eye contact	Recorded facial expressions	Recorded use of hands	Recorded use of body language	Recorded vocal sounds	Recorded words	Notes
1	10	0	15	23	Frowning/sad expression; amazed expression; broad smile; expressive eyes	Took book	Calm body language throughout	Made a raspberry sound and an expression of "oh"	"Oh, darlin'" "Far" "How cute" "Look at that baby" "Oh look" "What is that here?" "Oh look at her"	Seemed more quickly and easily engaged viewing the book a second time. General good mood & attentive. Both appropriate & non-sensical verbalization. 10 min.
2	25	0	0	25	Smiled; inquisitive; face "lit-up"; sad; frowned; studied	x1 - pointed x2 - touched	0	0	*	Very verbal. Looked at photo. Commented, then lost interest until page turned. 15 min.
3	25	0	0	25	Giggling/laughter; mimicking	5x; turned pages a few times	Docile, pleasant	2	"Don't know, don't care"*	No children. Very conversant, perceptive. Developed relationship with facilitator. 10 min.
4	7	0	0	7	None recorded	2	Still	Words	"I don't care about it" "Take it" "Where's my husband?"	10 min.
5	6	0	0	6	None recorded	2	Very Mobile	Giggled several times	None other than to state, "I want my clothes & to leave"	Agitated. Distracted & difficult to engage both before and during. Short attention span. 5–10 min.
6	10; 1x post prompt	0	14	25	Generallly a flat affect; giggled at times; pensive/studied	With prompt	Calm	*Words used	*	No page turning or talking w/o prompt. 20-35 min.
7	9	2	3	13	Smiled; laughed; pensive; no response	x2 - pointed	Appeared distracted	Animated	*	Lots of stories, emotions, frustrations. Stopped abruptly. 20 min.

KEY

No. of minutes:	Total time that the person with dementia participated willingly with the photo book and/or facilitator.
Vocal sounds:	Generally anything that wasn't an articulated word.
Positive response:	A directed and emotionally engaged response.
Negative response:	An aversive or "pulling away" response.
Neutral response:	No overt response one way or the other, but not negative.
* :	Too much data to fit in chart. See narrative summary of research (p. 55).
Facilitator:	Person presenting book.